SOPHIE'S SUPER CIRCULATORY SYSTEM

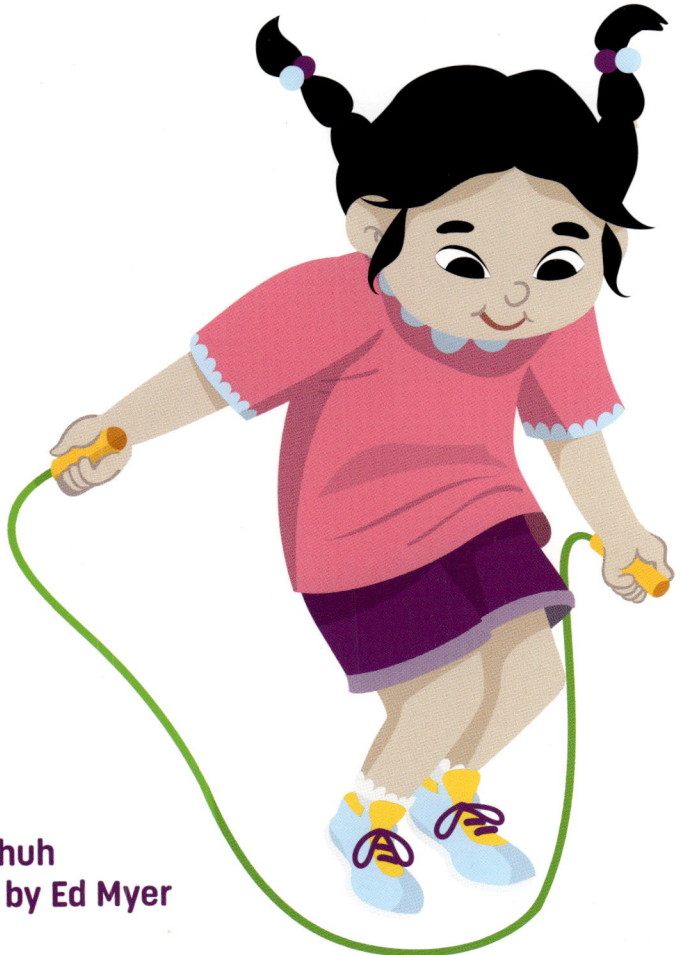

by Mari Schuh
illustrated by Ed Myer

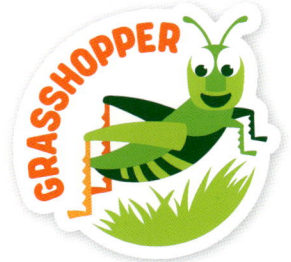

GRASSHOPPER

Tools for Parents & Teachers

Grasshopper Books enhance imagination and introduce the earliest readers to fiction with fun storylines and illustrations. The easy-to-read text supports early reading experiences with repetitive sentence patterns and sight words.

Before Reading

- Discuss the cover illustration. What do they see?

- Look at the glossary together. Discuss the words.

Read the Book

- Read the book to the child, or have him or her read independently.

- "Walk" through the book and look at the illustrations. Who is the main character? What is happening in the story?

After Reading

- Prompt the child to think more. Ask: How does your circulatory system help keep your body working?

Grasshopper Books are published by Jump!
5357 Penn Avenue South
Minneapolis, MN 55419
www.jumplibrary.com

Library of Congress Cataloging-in-Publication Data

Names: Schuh, Mari C., 1975– author.
Myer, Ed, illustrator.
Title: Sophie's super circulatory system / by Mari Schuh; illustrated by Ed Myer.
Description: Minneapolis, MN: Jump!, Inc., [2022]
Series: Let's look at body systems!
Includes index.
Audience: Ages 7-10
Identifiers: LCCN 2021038072 (print)
LCCN 2021038073 (ebook)
ISBN 9781636906560 (hardcover)
ISBN 9781636906577 (paperback)
ISBN 9781636906584 (ebook)
Subjects: LCSH: Cardiovascular system–Juvenile literature.
Heart–Juvenile literature.
Classification: LCC QP103 .S38 2022 (print)
LCC QP103 (ebook) | DDC 612.1–dc23
LC record available at https://lccn.loc.gov/2021038072
LC ebook record available at https://lccn.loc.gov/2021038073

Editor: Jenna Gleisner
Direction and Layout: Anna Peterson
Illustrator: Ed Myer

Printed in the United States of America at Corporate Graphics in North Mankato, Minnesota.

Table of Contents

Hardworking Heart 4

Where in the Body? 22

Let's Review! 23

To Learn More 23

Glossary 24

Index 24

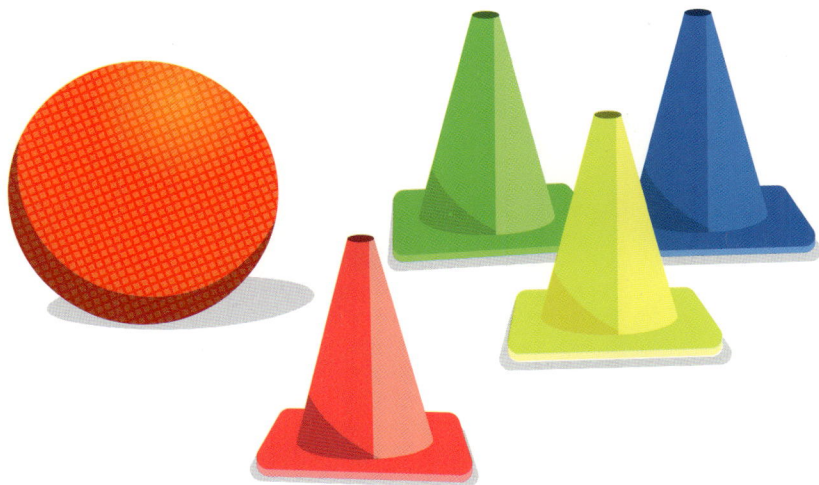

Hardworking Heart

"Way to go, class!" Ms. Collins says.
"Let's take a break."

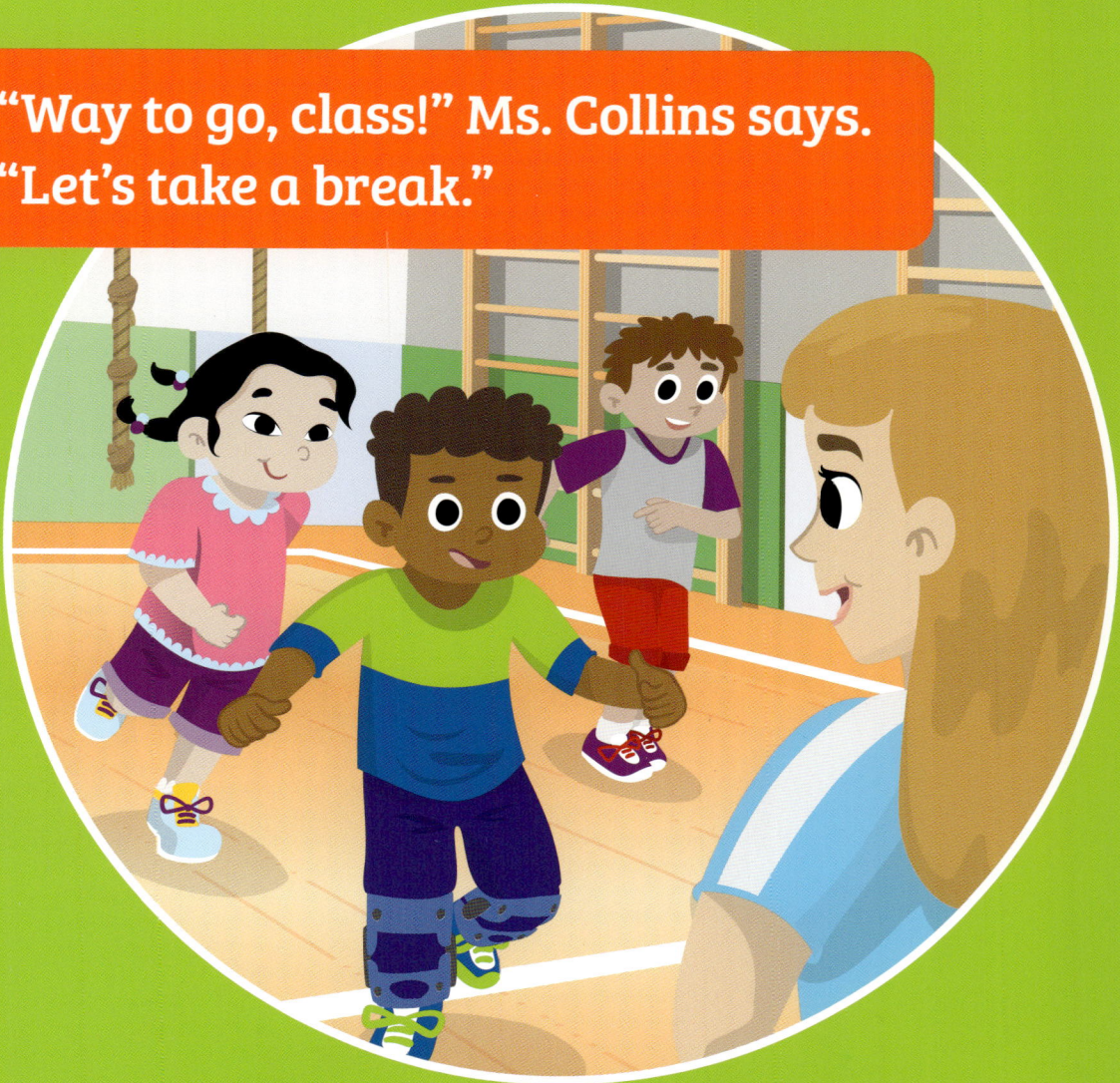

"That was fun!" Sophie says. "My heart is beating fast!"

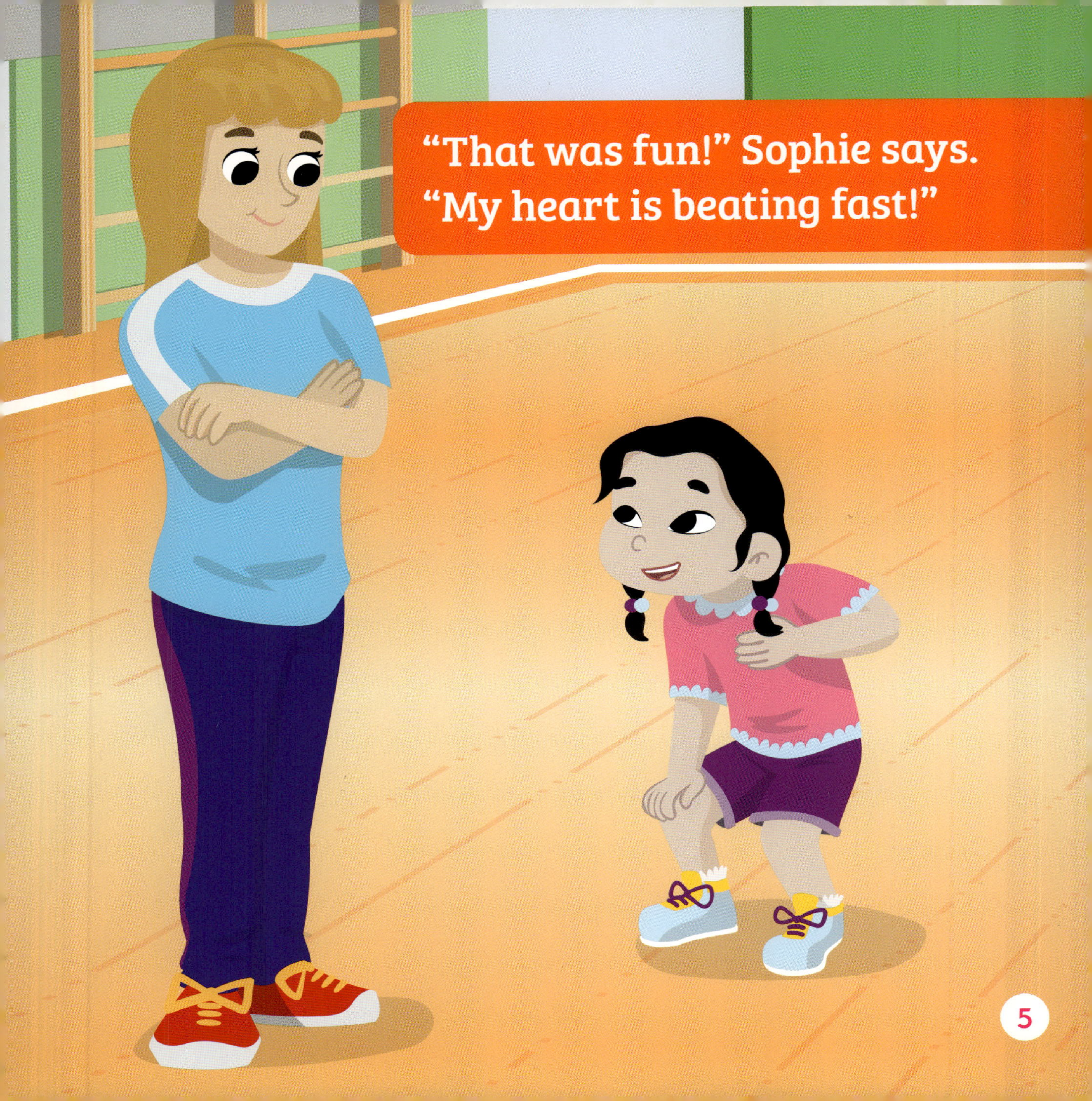

"Your heart is part of your circulatory system," says Ms. Collins. "It's busy pumping blood through a network of arteries, veins, and capillaries. These blood vessels bring oxygen and nutrients to your body so you have energy to play."

"Does my heart do that all the time? Or just when I exercise?" Sophie asks.

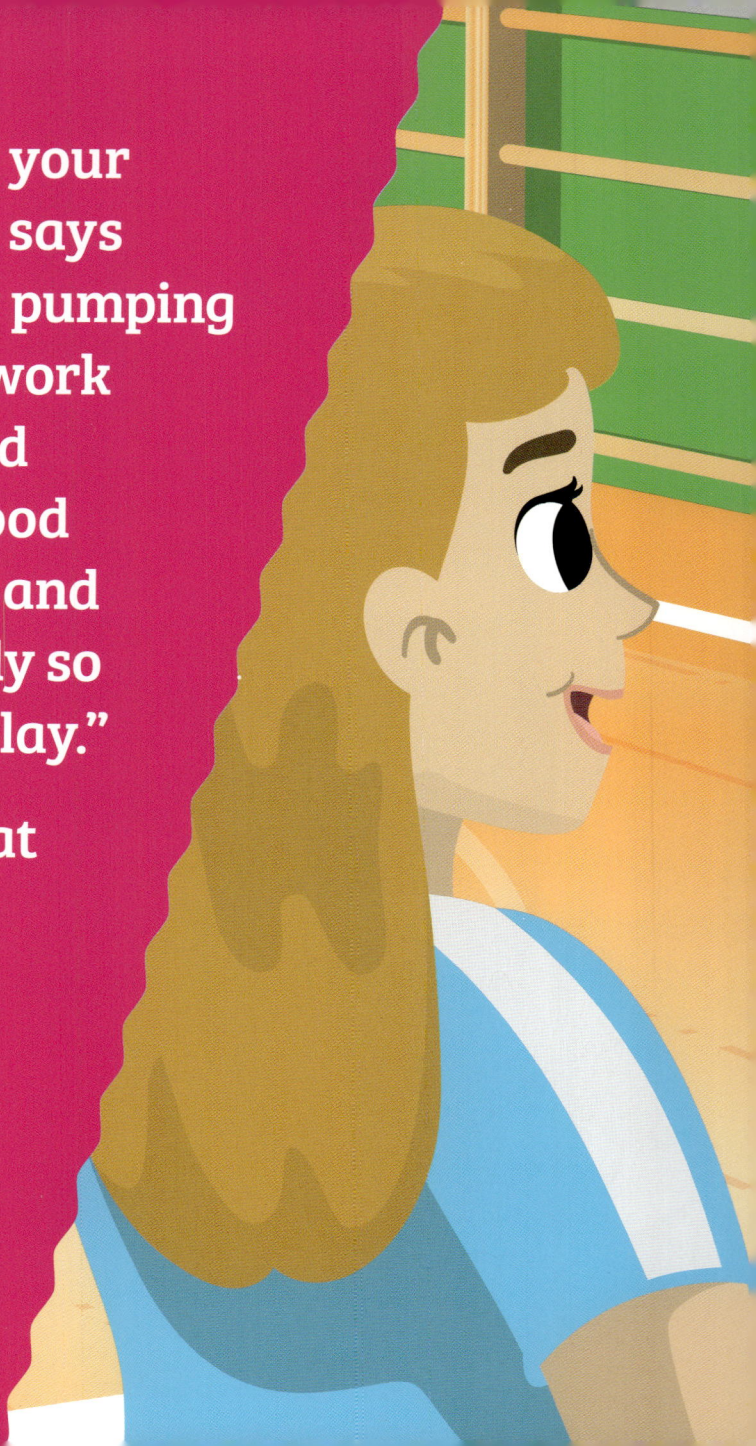

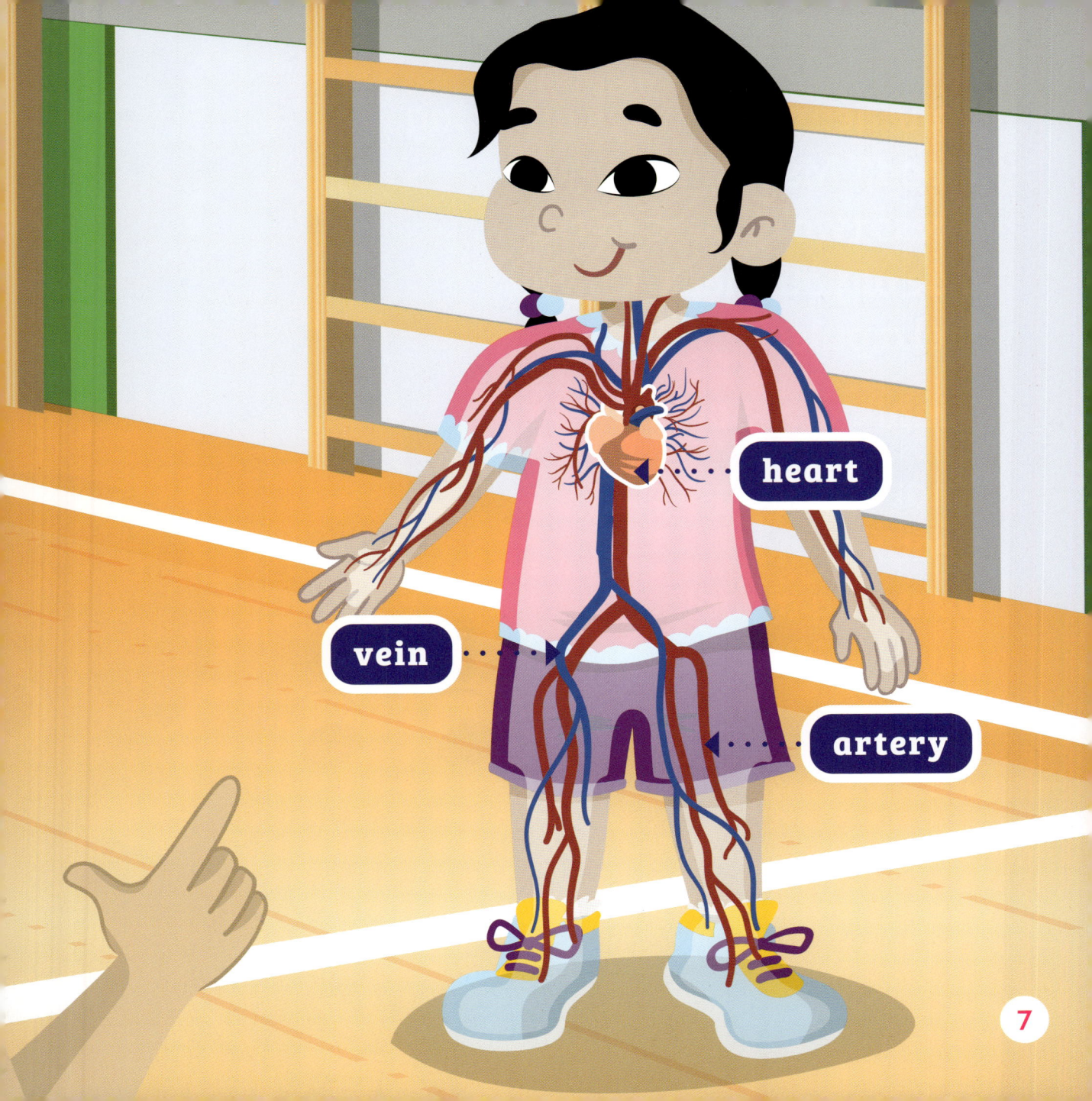

heart

vein

artery

"Your heart is always pumping blood," Ms. Collins says. "Press two fingers to the side of your neck. Do you feel a pulse?"

"Yeah!" says Sophie.

"That is your heart beating and pumping blood!" says Ms. Collins.

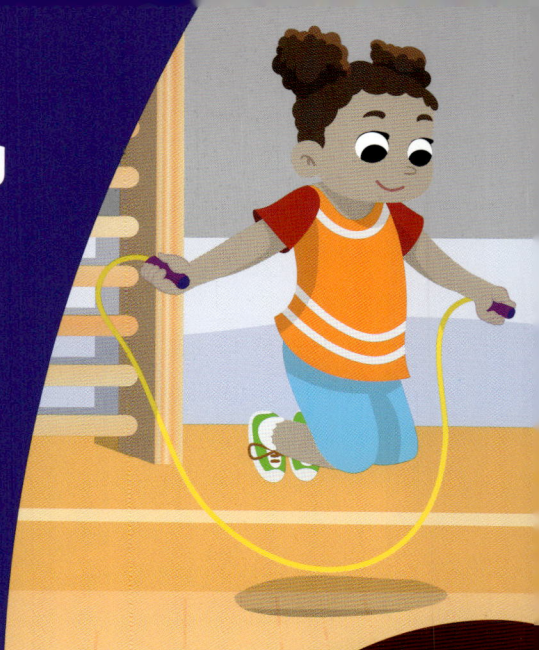

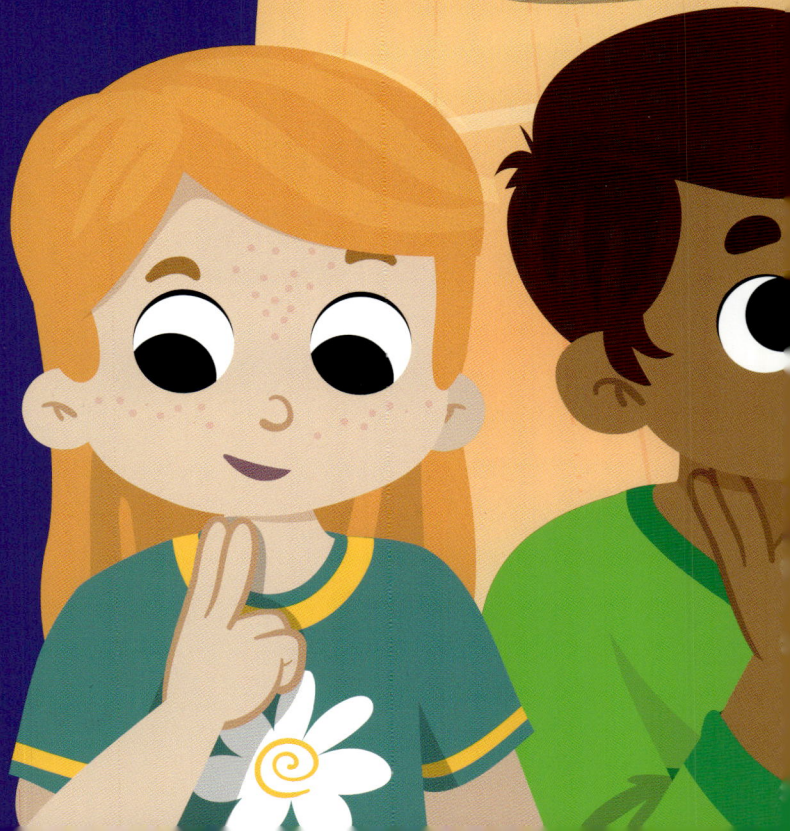

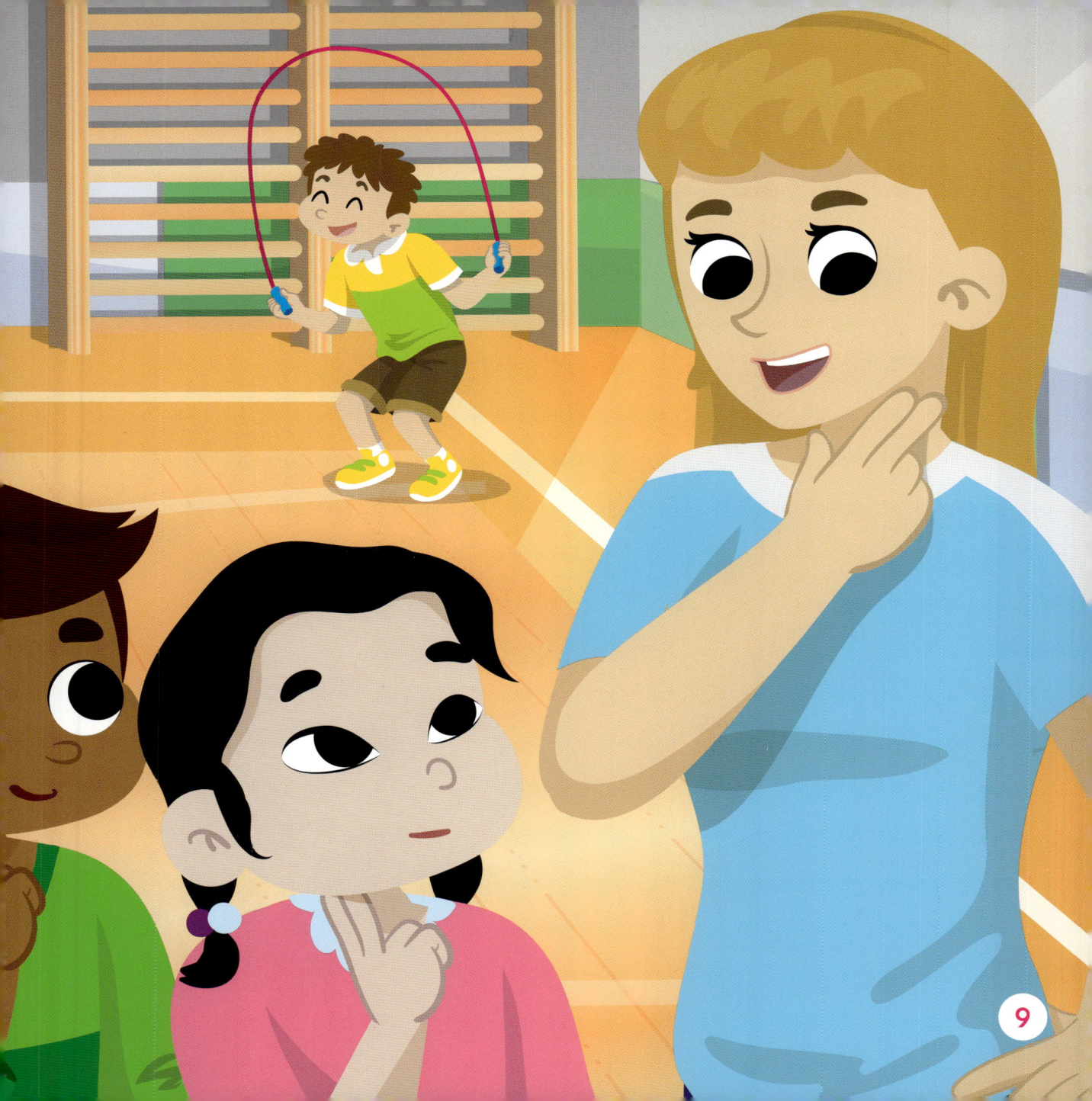

"Why does my heart beat faster when I exercise?" asks Sophie.

"So it can pump blood faster and deliver more oxygen to your body," Ms. Collins says.

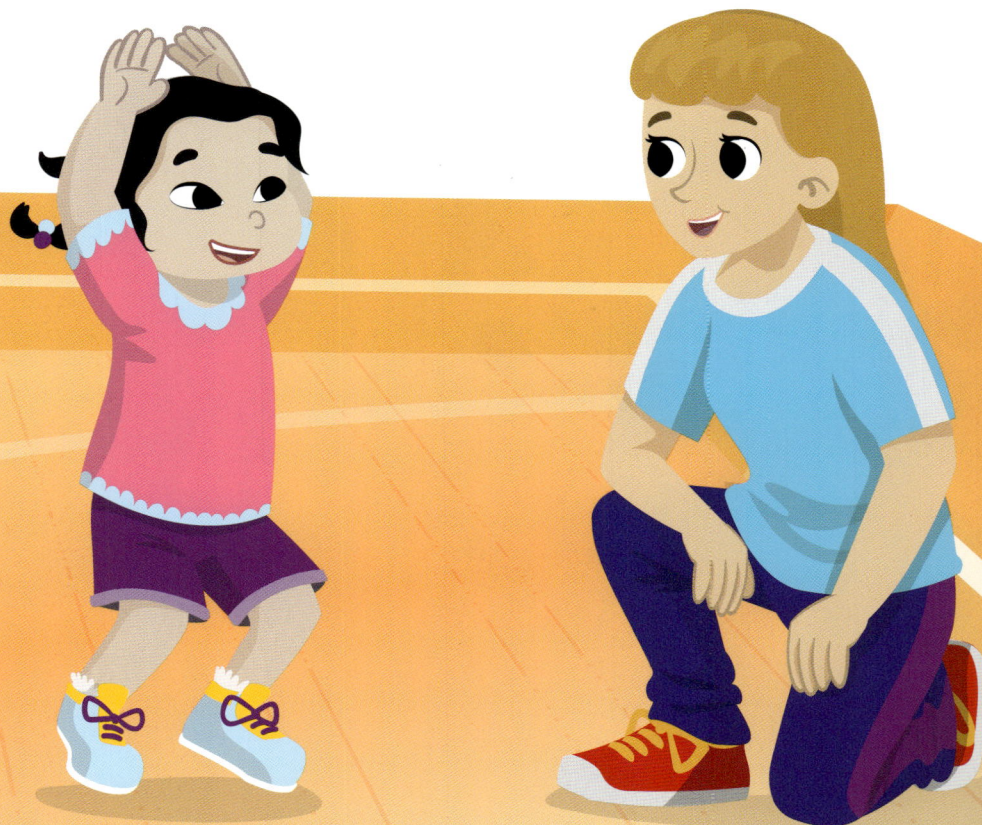

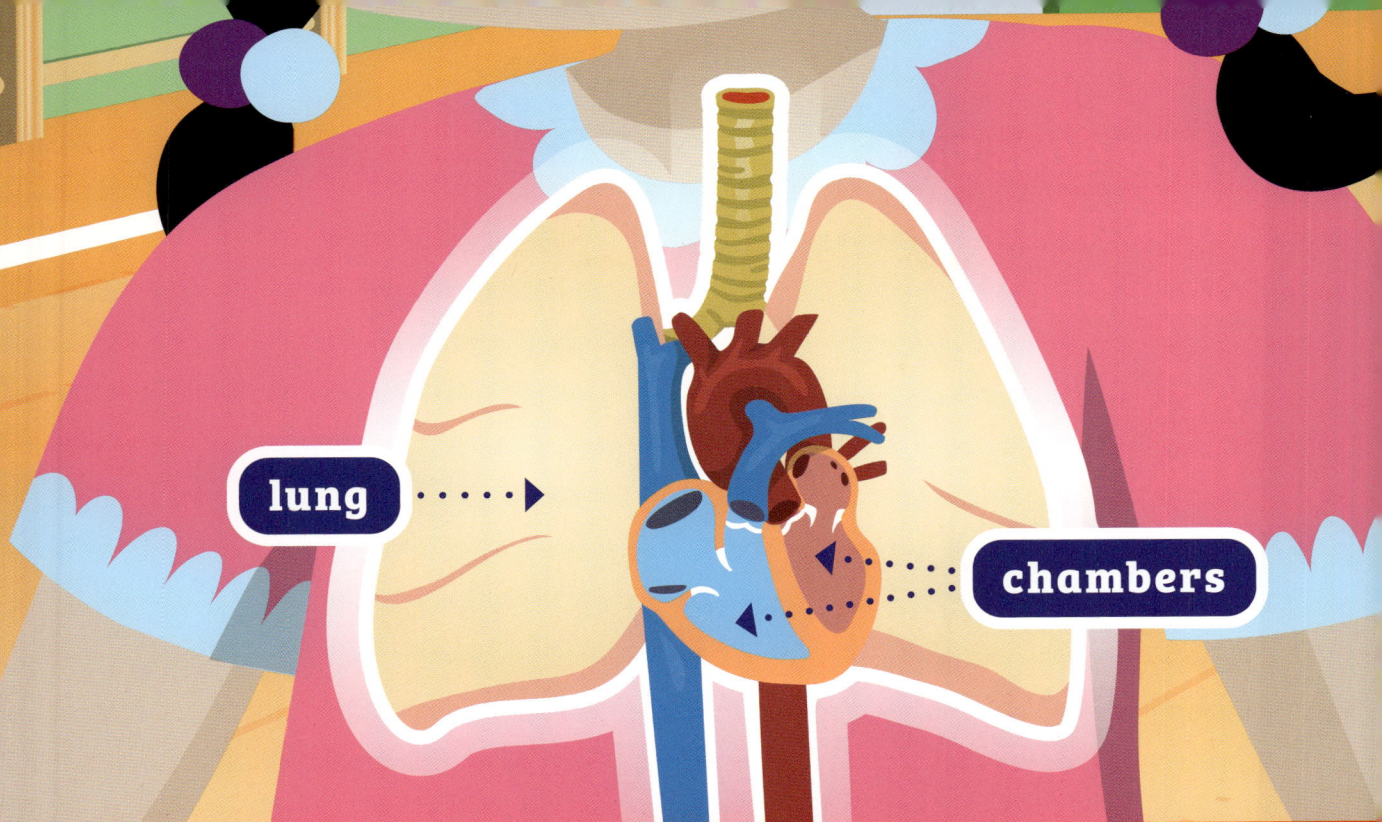

lung

chambers

"When you breathe in, oxygen goes into your lungs. It moves into your blood and heart. Your heart is made of strong muscle and has four chambers. These squeeze and relax to pump blood," Ms. Collins continues.

"How does blood move around my body?" asks Sophie.

"Arteries carry blood that's full of oxygen away from the heart and to the rest of the body. Veins carry blood that needs oxygen back to the heart," says Ms. Collins.

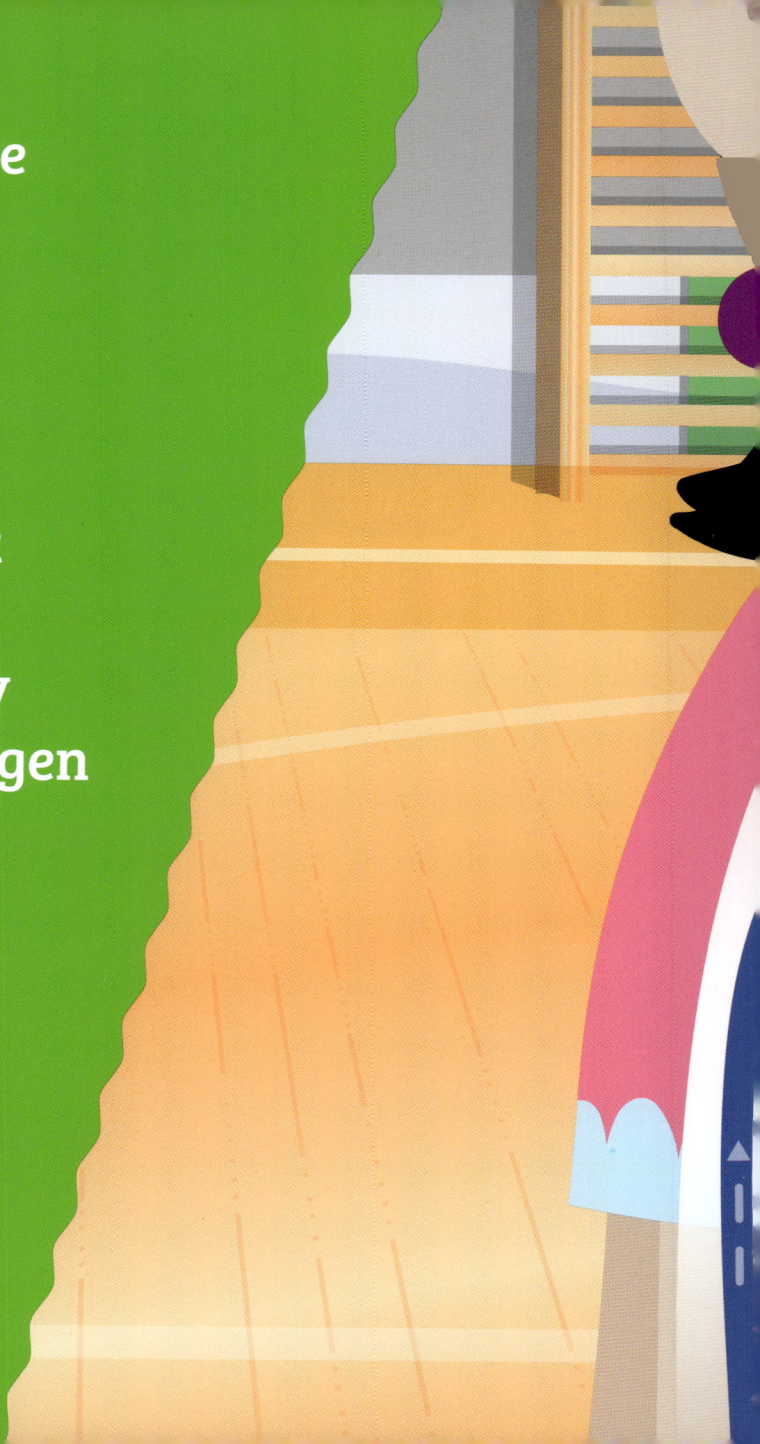

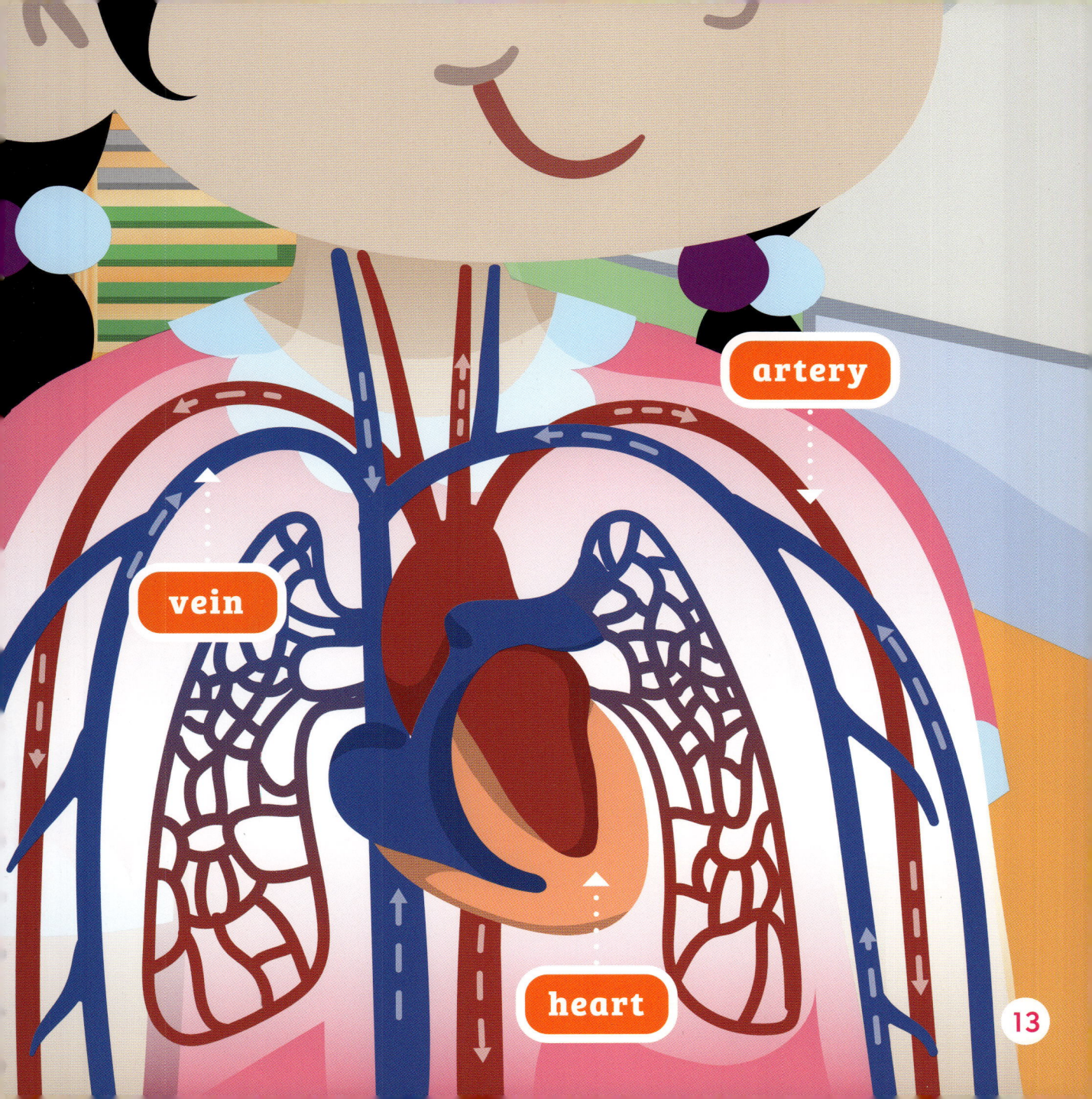

artery

vein

heart

13

"You can see your veins in your arms. Look," says Ms. Collins.

"But blood is red. Why do my veins look blue?" Sophie asks.

"That's just how light travels through your skin," Ms. Collins says.

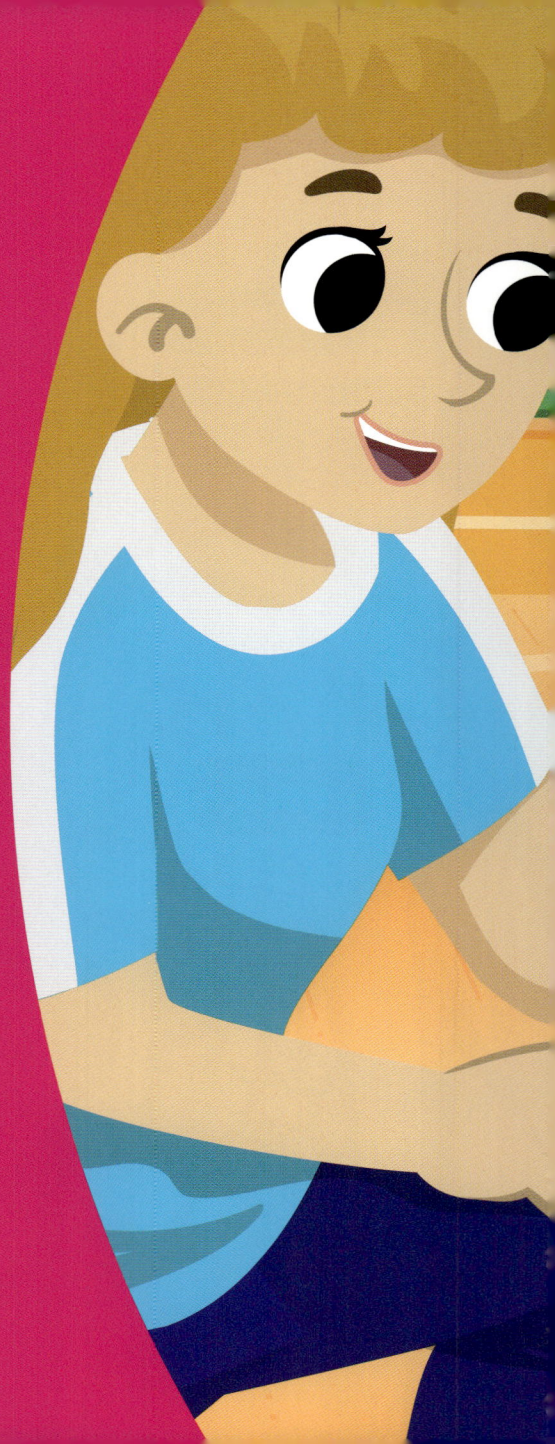

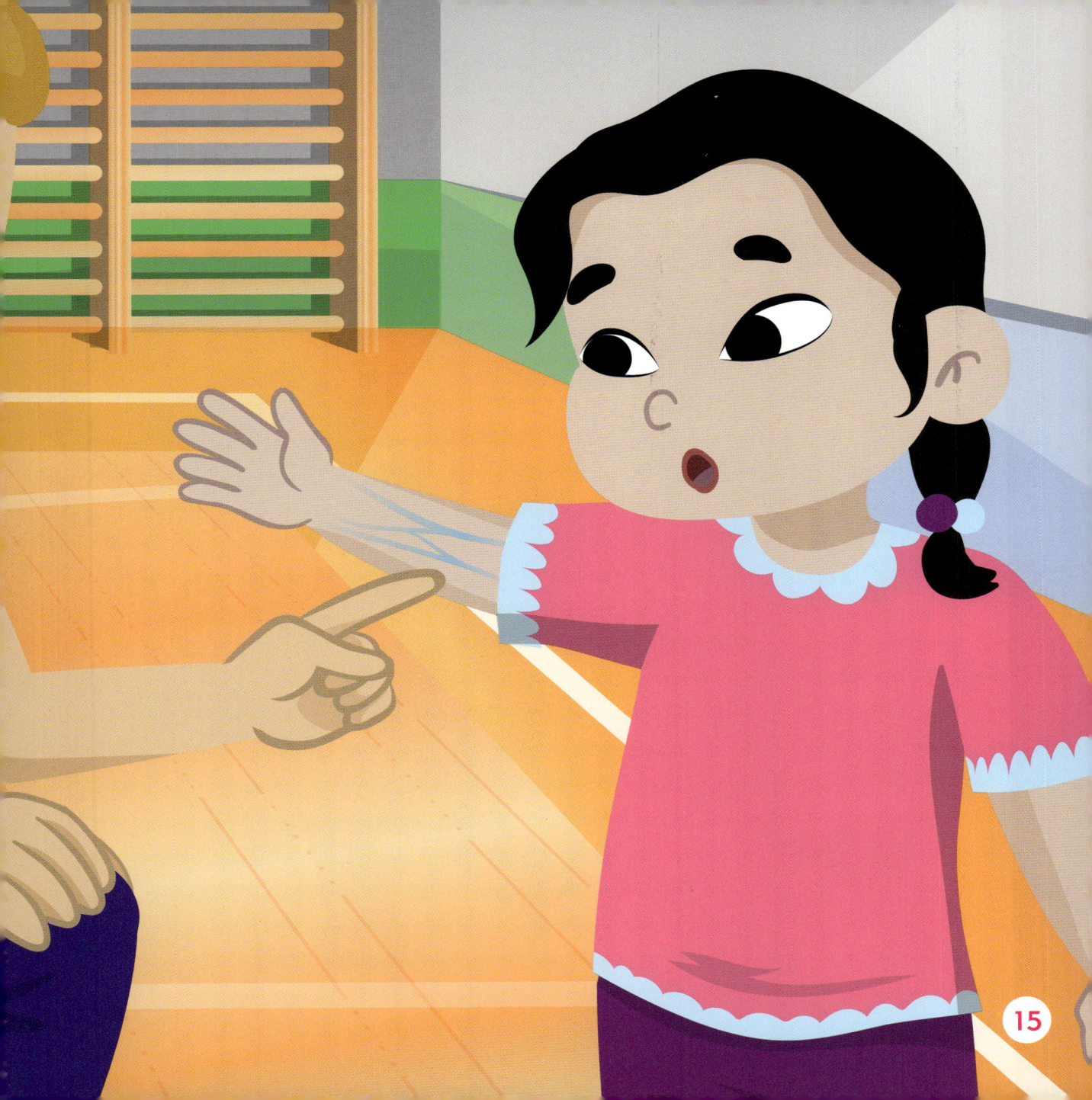

"Your muscles, organs, and cells need oxygen to work. Your blood brings oxygen to them," says Ms. Collins.

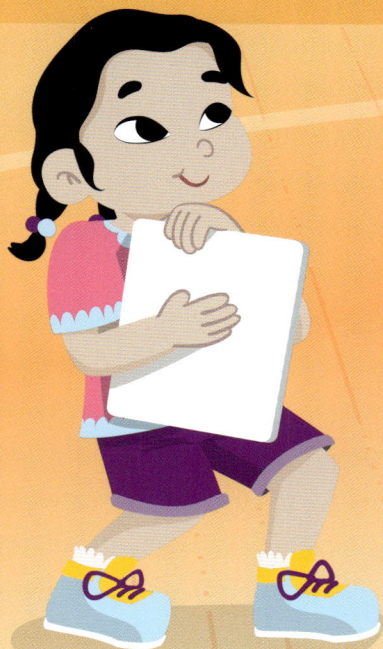

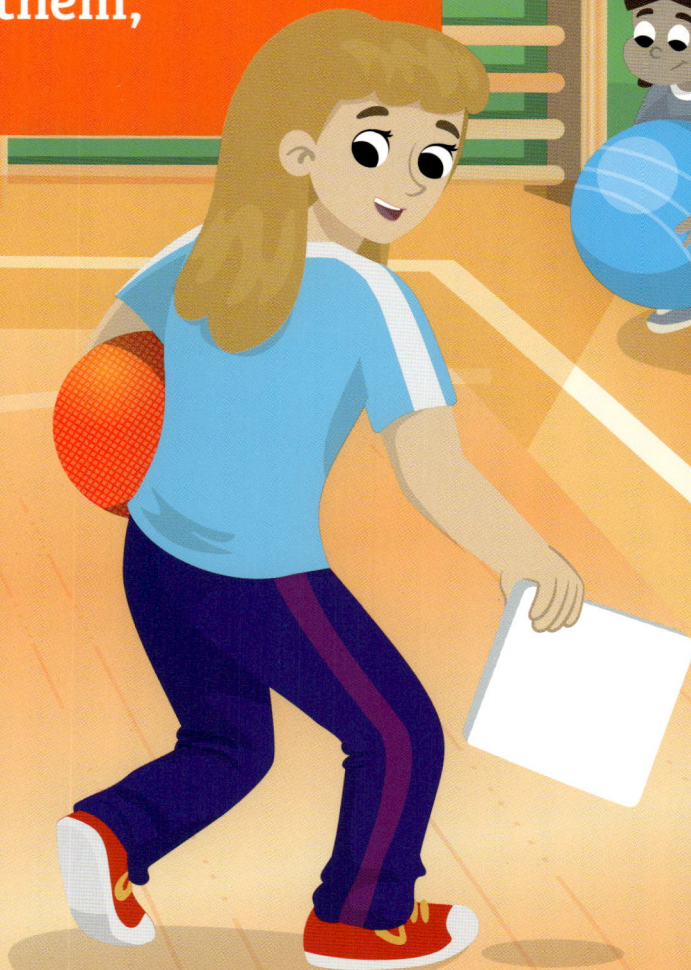

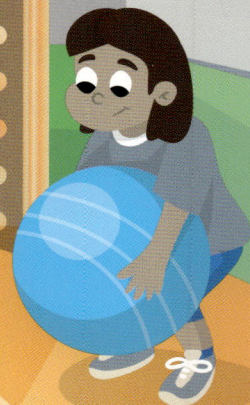

capillaries

"How does my blood get to them?" Sophie asks.

"Blood flows into capillaries. Oxygen and nutrients move out of your blood and into your cells," says Ms. Collins.

17

"So what is my circulatory system doing right now?" Sophie asks.

"Your cells are using oxygen and making carbon dioxide. Your veins carry blood back to your heart. The blood goes to your lungs to get more oxygen. You breathe out the carbon dioxide. Then you breathe in oxygen, and it all starts over again!" Ms. Collins answers.

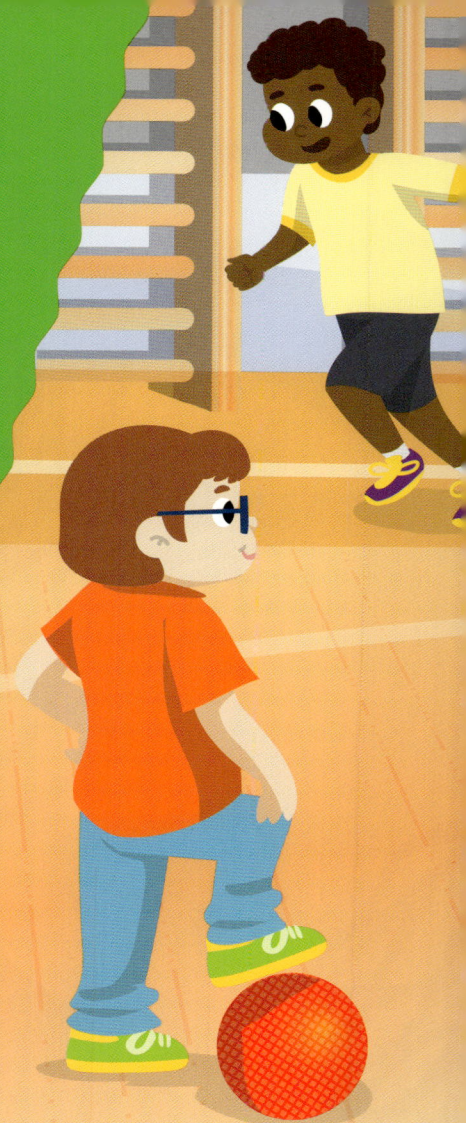

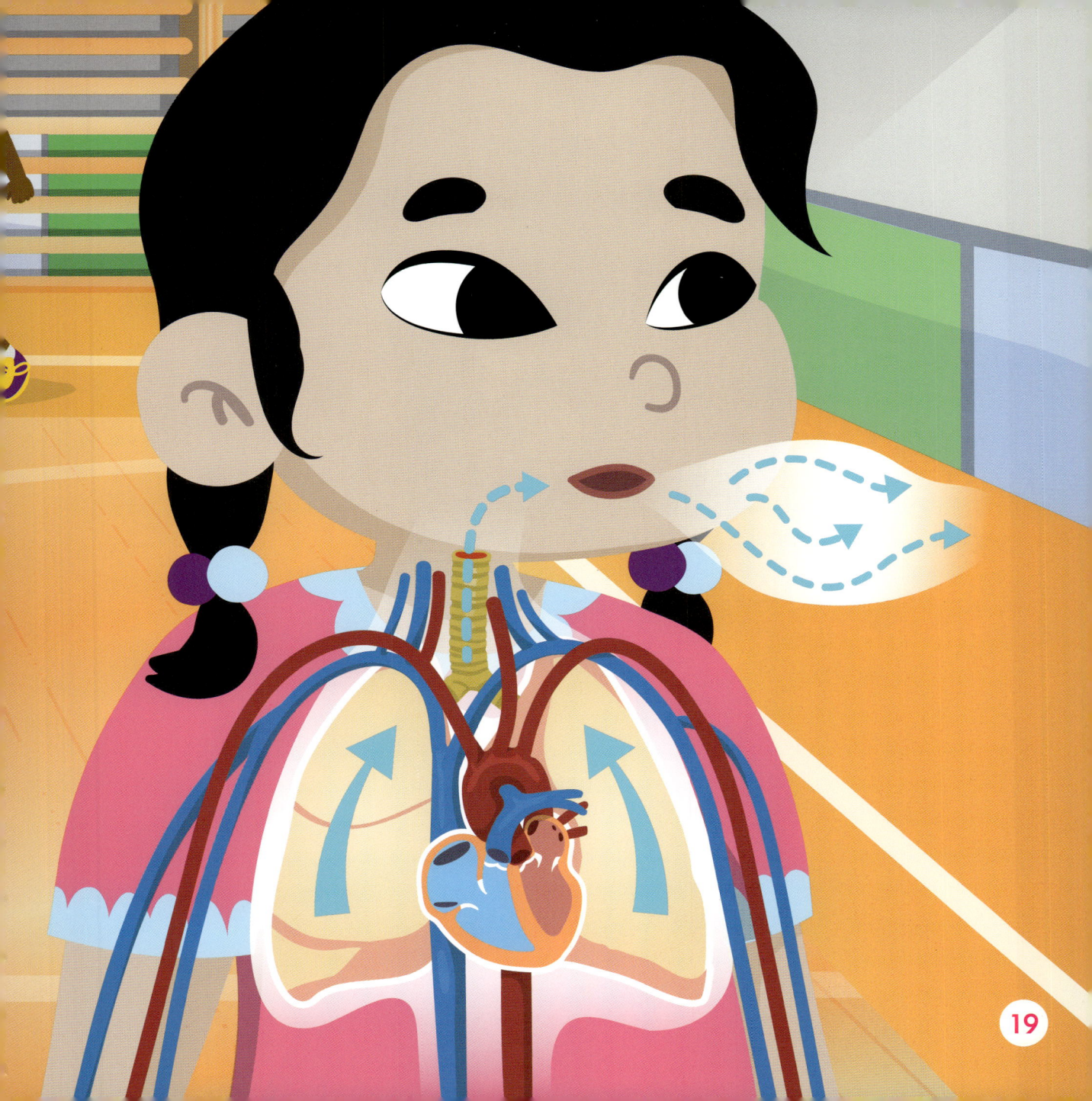

"I play every day," Sophie says. "My circulatory system must be super strong!"

"That's great, Sophie!" Ms. Collins says. "Exercise keeps your heart strong. A strong heart is better at pumping blood. Now let's play some kickball!"

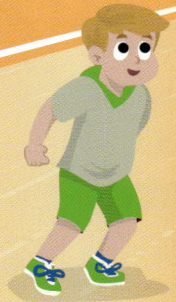

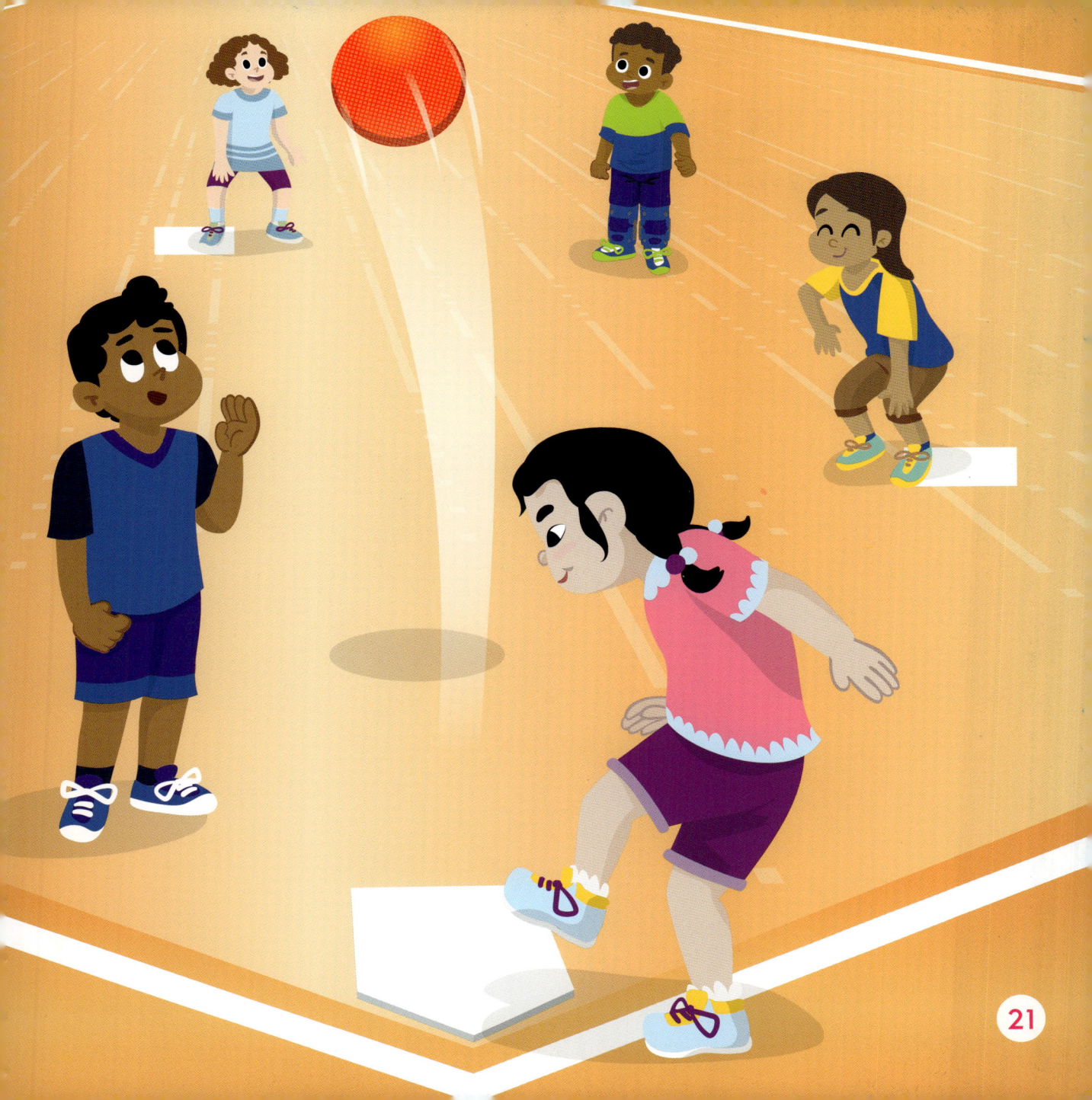

Where in the Body?

The circulatory system carries blood throughout the body. Take a look!

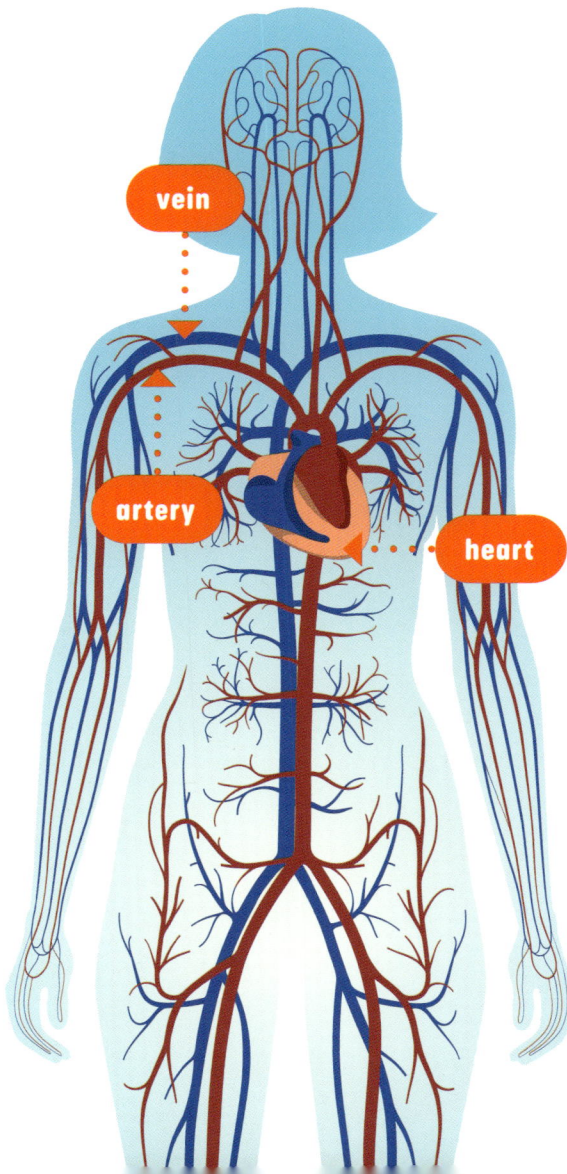

vein

artery

heart

Let's Review!

The circulatory system includes a network of blood vessels. What are the three types of blood vessels?

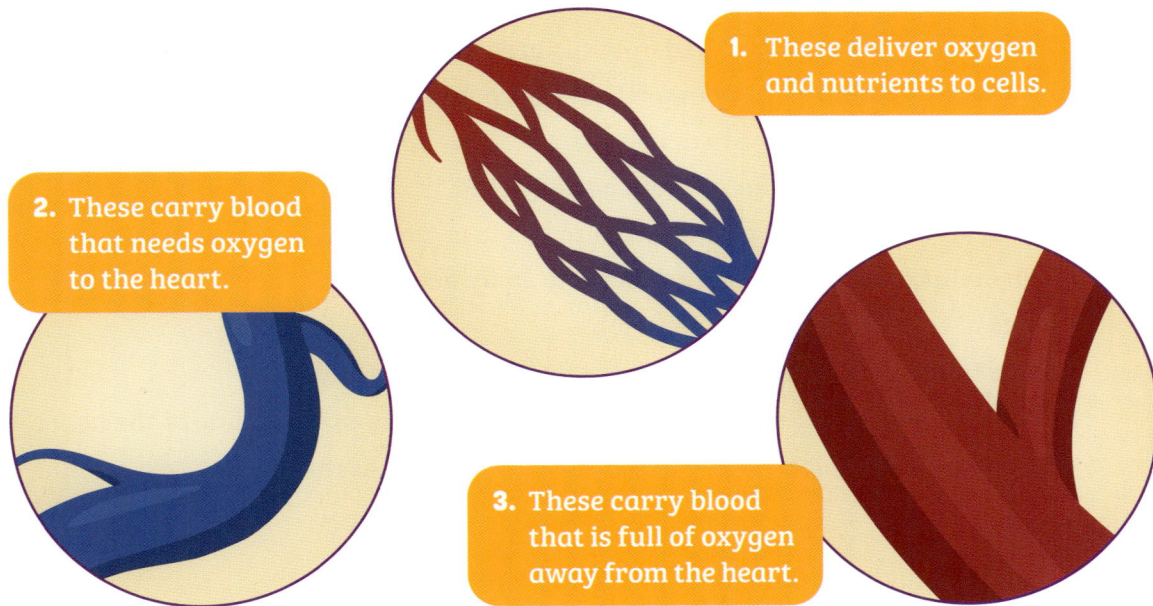

1. These deliver oxygen and nutrients to cells.

2. These carry blood that needs oxygen to the heart.

3. These carry blood that is full of oxygen away from the heart.

To Learn More

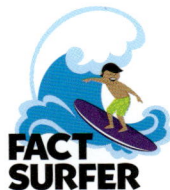

Finding more information is as easy as 1, 2, 3.

FACT SURFER

1. Go to www.factsurfer.com
2. Enter "**Sophie'ssupercirculatorysystem**" into the search box.
3. Choose your book to see a list of websites.

Glossary

arteries: Vessels that carry blood from your heart to the rest of your body.

blood vessels: Tubes in your body through which blood flows.

capillaries: Small vessels that transfer blood between arteries and veins.

carbon dioxide: A gas that humans and animals breathe out.

cells: The smallest parts of living things. A microscope is needed to see cells.

chambers: Enclosed spaces in the heart.

energy: The strength to do things without getting tired.

muscle: Tissue in the body that can contract to produce movement.

nutrients: Proteins, minerals, and vitamins your body needs to stay healthy and strong.

organs: Parts of the body that do certain jobs.

oxygen: A gas found in the air, which humans need to breathe and live.

pulse: A regular, rhythmic throbbing caused by the squeezing and relaxing of the heart.

veins: Vessels that carry blood to the heart from other parts of the body.

Index

arteries 6, 12

beating 5, 8, 10

blood 6, 8, 10, 11, 12, 14, 16, 17, 18, 20

capillaries 6, 17

carbon dioxide 18

cells 16, 17, 18

energy 6

exercise 6, 10, 20

heart 5, 6, 8, 10, 11, 12, 18, 20

lungs 11, 18

muscle 11, 16

nutrients 6, 17

organs 16

oxygen 6, 10, 11, 12, 16, 17, 18

pulse 8

veins 6, 12, 14, 18